YOUR KNOWLEDGE HAS VALUE

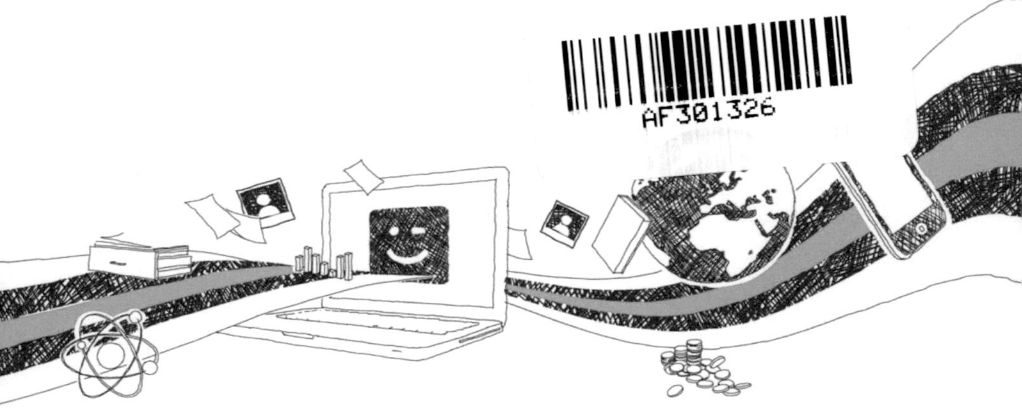

- We will publish your bachelor's and master's thesis, essays and papers

- Your own eBook and book - sold worldwide in all relevant shops

- Earn money with each sale

Upload your text at www.GRIN.com and publish for free

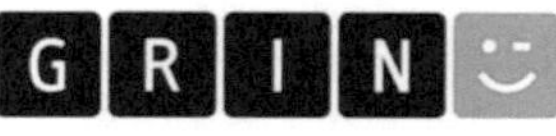

Imprint:

Copyright © 2009 GRIN Verlag, Open Publishing GmbH
Print and binding: Books on Demand GmbH, Norderstedt Germany
ISBN: 9783640598199

Charlotte Wilkinson

Fetal Alcohol Syndrome/Effects

GRIN Publishing

Fetal Alcohol Syndrome/Effects

A Research Paper

Charlotte Wilkinson
11/30/2009

Fetal Alcohol Syndrome (FAS) is a part of Fetal Alcohol Spectrum Disorder, and is also referred to as Fetal Alcohol Effects. However, FAS is the clinical diagnosis term for any one on the spectrum. So for the purposes of this paper, it will be referred to as such. FAS is one of the leading causes of preventable birth defects and developmental delays (Graefe, 2003). It is a form of brain injury caused by alcohol usage by the mother during pregnancy, and is more prevalent in our world than many people are aware of. 9 out of every 1000 births are FAS births (Knowledge Network 2009), and as many as 1 in 4 births may have had alcohol exposure, but no noticeable effects. There is no association between *paternal* alcohol consumption and birth outcome (Saskatchewan Institute on Prevention of Handicaps, 2000). Contributing factors to the cause of FAS include malnutrition, other drug usage, already having a child with FAS, and having a history of substance abuse. It is not genetic or inherited (Graefe, 2003).

The effects of FAS show themselves in many ways: physically, emotionally, and intellectually. Depending on where the child is on the spectrum, they may have facial abnormalities, or they may not. There is no complete diagnosis for FAS – how the child is affected is mostly dependent on what time during fetal development the mother drank and how much alcohol was consumed. The impact of the alcohol on the fetus also depends on the pattern of consumption (regular vs. binge) as well as the genetic makeup and tolerance of the mother and the fetus (SIPH, 2000). Alcohol changes the way the brain processes and responds, therefore a child who has FAS will not respond or process in the same way as someone who does not. There is no safe amount of alcohol to drink during pregnancy, and there is no cure for FAS.

Diagnosis of FAS often goes unnoticed, especially if the effects are not visible, and many children aren't diagnosed until they reach school-age if they are diagnosed at all. According to the Saskatchewan Institute of Handicap Prevention, 1 out of every 100 children born is suffering from some sort of Fetal Alcohol Effects (2000). It can be incredibly frustrating for an FAS affected individual to go without a diagnosis, because this means that they automatically get labeled as stupid, or a problem. Their peers and caregivers can, without proper knowledge of FAS, assume that they are acting up deliberately, when in fact it is that their brain just can't process that their behaviour is unacceptable (Knowledge Network, 2009). Early diagnosis is possible by a medical doctor, but only with parental consent. Once that is obtained, the child is given a physical exam and a thorough history is taken. It is possible for FAS to be diagnosed without knowledge of the mother's alcohol consumption, as long as all other characteristics are present (SIPH, 2000). Early diagnosis assists teachers, caregivers, and parents to know what to expect and plan accordingly. It also allows the possibility for secondary disabilities, which will be addressed later in the paper, to be prevented (SIPH, 2000).

Facial abnormalities in an FAS child include a small eye opening, flat thin upper lip, little or no groove between nose and lip, short nose, flat mid face, and minor ear abnormalities. Other physical characteristics of FAS include small head size at birth, structural abnormalities in the brain, poor fine motor skills, poor hand eye coordination, poor gait when walking, hearing loss not related to injury or illness, low birth weight, weight loss not due to poor nutrition, and low weight to height rate (SIPH, 2000).

Physically is not the only way that FAS affects a person. It also affects them emotionally and intellectually. Often, an FAS-affected individual can be younger intellectually than they are physically. It is a brain disorder, and it is not always visible on the face or body, making it very often an invisible disability. In *Fetal Alcohol Syndrome: A resource for professonials, Let's find a solution,* which was written by the Saskatchewan Institute on Prevention of Handicaps (SIPH), the authors lay it out by age groups, and list the intellectual and emotional affects and challenges FAS has on a person from infancy through adulthood.

As an infant/toddler (ages 0-5 according to SIPH), an FAS –affected child can be overwhelmed by stimuli which can lead to hiding somewhere and refusing to come out. They have difficulty establishing routine, following directions , obeying rules, may have frequent temper tantrums, and become distracted and hyperactive more easily than others. In the school years (ages 6-11), the child is easily influenced by others, has difficulty understanding the consequences of their actions, may show signs of delayed cognitive and physical development, has poor impulse control, may continue to have temper tantrums, has difficulty separating fantasy from reality, and has difficulty with social situations. FAS affected children get frustrated and angry easier than non-FAS affected children, and this can have a huge impact on their social situations and who befriends them (SIPH, 2000).

By the time the FAS affected child is an adolescent (12-18) they usually have increased negative behaviour (stealing, tantrums, etc),faulty logic , continuing struggles with not understanding consequences of their actions, increased depression and low self-esteem, and are often behind academically. This is quite often due to the lack of the fine motor skills set. Some children can't write their names when they first enter school, due to this missing skill set, which then sets them behind academically all their lives. FAS-affected individuals struggle with it their whole lives. It is a lifelong disability. By the time they have reached the age of adulthood (18+), while some may think the challenges will end, there is actually a whole new set of challenges the individual has to deal with. They have continued difficulty in social situations, difficulty finding and keeping a job, and also must contend with depression and withdrawal from others. This is also the stage at which many individuals leave home and go to college or out on their own, which proves to be an even more difficult transition for the FAS affected individual. Secondary disabilities that can happen as a result of FAS, and can occur at any stage, include learning problems, drug abuse, and mental health issues (SIPH, 2000). An FAS diagnosis is often overlapped with diagnosis of other developmental disabilities, which include ADD, Attachment Disorder, Oppositional Defiant Disorder, Conduct Disorder , and Autism (Graefe, 2003). This therefore means that knowledge of those disabilities is valuable to know along with knowledge of FAS, so as to understand as best as possible where the child is coming from and how to best support and help them.

Prevention of FAS is fairly simple, but easier said than done. Don't drink when you are pregnant.

No amount of alcohol is safe on a fetus, as this paper has outlined. That being said, 50% of pregnancies

are unplanned, and if a woman doesn't know she is pregnant and has a drink or two, these can and will

affect the fetus (Knowledge Network, 2009). This is part of the reason why it goes unnoticed. However,

if a woman finds out she is pregnant, she can stop drinking immediately to prevent any further damage.

Or, if she suspects she might be pregnant, she could choose to refrain from drinking until she knows for

sure.

An FAS-affected individual will be affected by it their whole life, as mentioned above. They

hopefully have many support systems and people around them to help them deal with their condition. It

is vitally important that, at some point in the child's life, when the effects start to show themselves, the

parent talks to the child about their FAS, and what that means for them. The parent or guardian must be

sure to be clear with the child that it is not the child's fault, these things just happen. There are many

things professionals and parents can do when working with FAS kids to aid in helping them through and

helping them to live fulfilling lives that we all know they can. Some of these things include: providing a

safe, stable, nurturing environment for them at all times; having psychological, educational, and

behaviour evaluations; using clear, concrete consequences for behaviour ; monitoring their health,

sexual activity, and social environment; making sure they don't get over-stimulated; having a routine,

consistency, and giving reminders (SIPH, 2000). This is particularly important once they have reached

the school age and their routine changes. An easy way to think about what FAS affected children need is

to remember the 4S's and C: structure, supervision, simplicity, steps, and context (Graefe, 2003).

Keeping it as consistent as possible with the same routine at home is essential for the FAS-affected child,

as it helps them to not get as frustrated and angry. Other ways to aid in this concept include being

specific when giving directions, being brief and keeping directions short, using visual cues and expressive

gestures, limiting distractions, reminders, linking tasks together, and helping them to interpret others cues (Graefe, 2003). As well, make sure that when the child is misbehaving to separate the child from the behaviour itself; try and intervene before the inappropriate behaviour escalates; designate a place for quiet time, and don't forget the positive acknowledgement when the child does as asked, or changes their behaviour! (Graefe, 2003).The parent or professional living with an FAS affected individual does not have it easy either. They must remember their own needs, and other ways to make it easier on both parties include: adapting to the child's environment, not the other way around; providing respite care if the parent doesn't have help so the caregiver can get a break; educating the community about FAS and the affect it has on children; and advocating for the child (SIPH, 2000). As mentioned before, without a diagnosis, the child will get labeled as a problem child, or as stupid, among other things. People will talk, and people will get frustrated. Advocating for a child is doing everything within one's power to get them the help they need to live rewarding, fulfilling lives. This is helped by the fact that more people are becoming aware of FAS and its affect on children's behaviour. That number will hopefully increase with more education and awareness about FAS.

FAS-affected children *can* lead normal, fulfilling lives when given the right kind of support, guidance, structure, consistency and patience to help them with the tools they need to be successful. There are many positive characteristics of FAS, all of which can help the individual lead a satisfying life. These characteristics include: great imaginations, creative, a deep sense of fairness and a strong sense of self, friendly, affectionate, a love for children and animals, sensitive, curious, loyal, trusting, rich fantasy life, exceptional long term memory, and spontaneous (Graefe, 2003). As one of the FAS affected girls in the video *"Finding Hope, Fetal Alcohol Spectrum Disorder"* (Knowledge Network, 2009), said: "people don't choose to have a bad day because of a brain disorder".

References

Graefe, S. (2003) *Living with FASD: A Guide for Parents* , Toronto, ON. Society of Special Needs
    Adoptive Parents

Saskatchewan Institute on Prevention of Handicaps (2000), *Fetal Alcohol Syndrome: A Resource for
    Professionals, Let's find a solution*. Saskatoon, SK

Knowledge Network (Producer), British Columbia Ministry of Children & Family Development
    (Producer), PLEA Community Society of British Columbia (Producer). (2009) *Finding Hope: Fetal
    Alcohol Spectrum Disorder* [DVD]. Canada: Force Four Entertainment

YOUR KNOWLEDGE HAS VALUE

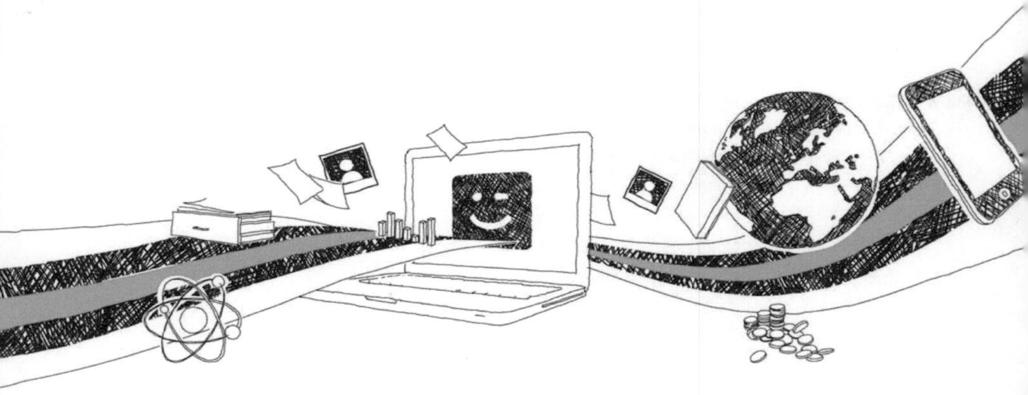

- We will publish your bachelor's and
  master's thesis, essays and papers

- Your own eBook and book -
  sold worldwide in all relevant shops

- Earn money with each sale

Upload your text at www.GRIN.com
and publish for free

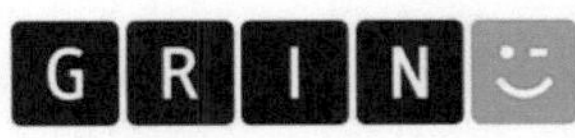